YOUR KNOWLEDGE HAS VALUE

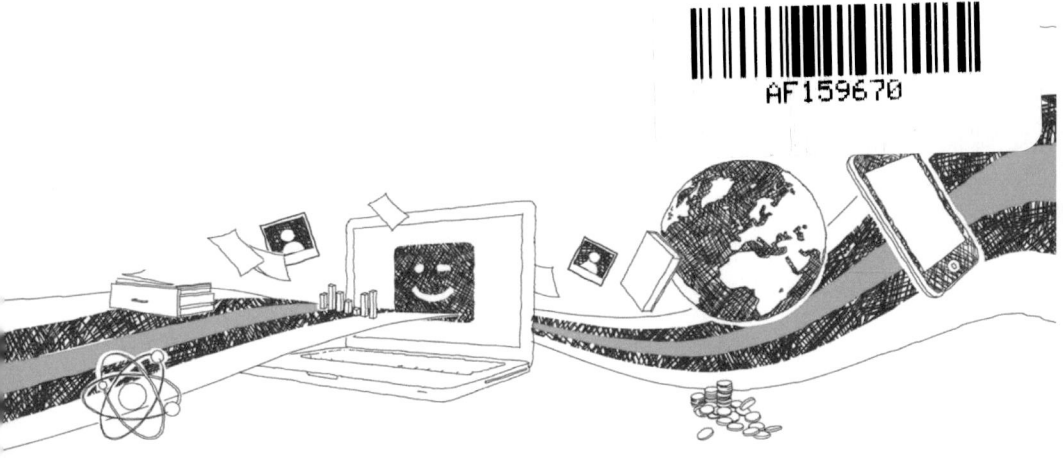

- We will publish your bachelor's and master's thesis, essays and papers

- Your own eBook and book - sold worldwide in all relevant shops

- Earn money with each sale

Upload your text at www.GRIN.com and publish for free

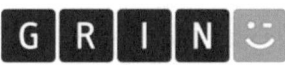

Bibliographic information published by the German National Library:

The German National Library lists this publication in the National Bibliography; detailed bibliographic data are available on the Internet at http://dnb.dnb.de .

This book is copyright material and must not be copied, reproduced, transferred, distributed, leased, licensed or publicly performed or used in any way except as specifically permitted in writing by the publishers, as allowed under the terms and conditions under which it was purchased or as strictly permitted by applicable copyright law. Any unauthorized distribution or use of this text may be a direct infringement of the author s and publisher s rights and those responsible may be liable in law accordingly.

Imprint:

Copyright © 2016 GRIN Verlag, Open Publishing GmbH
Print and binding: Books on Demand GmbH, Norderstedt Germany
ISBN: 9783668371606

This book at GRIN:

http://www.grin.com/en/e-book/349844/main-challenges-faced-by-local-health-managers-in-times-of-economic-crisis

Bruce Wembulua Shinga

Main challenges faced by local health managers in times of economic crisis

GRIN Publishing

GRIN - Your knowledge has value

Since its foundation in 1998, GRIN has specialized in publishing academic texts by students, college teachers and other academics as e-book and printed book. The website www.grin.com is an ideal platform for presenting term papers, final papers, scientific essays, dissertations and specialist books.

Visit us on the internet:

http://www.grin.com/

http://www.facebook.com/grincom

http://www.twitter.com/grin_com

In dem folgenden Essay möchte ich mich mit einem politischen System befassen, das die chinesische Gesellschaft in den letzten 30 Jahren sowohl geistig als auch demographisch stark beeinflusst hat und international immer wieder für Diskussionen sorgt: Die Ein-Kind-Politik. Sie stellt einen großen Eingriff in die Privatsphäre der Menschen dar, welcher allerdings allgemein akzeptiert wird – zum Wohle des Landes. (…)

The main challenges faced by local health managers in times of economic crisis.

Dr WEMBULUA SHINGA BRUCE

Student of online Master of Science in Health Management

UNIVERSITÀ TELEMATICA INTERNAZIONALE UNINETTUNO.

This piece of work describe succinctly what a health services manager often faces in times of economic crisis

Academic year 2016 -2017

Contents

INTRODUCTION 3

CHAP. 1 : IMPACTS OF AN ECONOMIC CRISIS TO A LOCAL SOCIETY 4

CHAP. 2: MAIN MANAGERIAL CHALLENGES IN TIMES OF ECONOMIC CRISIS 6

CONCLUSION 7

BIBLIOGRAPHY 9

INTRODUCTION

Almost nothing in our modern healthcare system is preserved from both immediate and long term effects of economic oscillations. The healthcare becomes more and more subject to higher technologies with a growing number of private, well organized and benefit - oriented hospitals. Researchers found that approximately 50% of health improvements were due to access to better technology, whereas remaining gains resulted from income improvements and better education. Healthcare is actually referenced to as one of the most complex, costly and challenged sector of our contemporary societies (Merson, Black and Mills 2012; Lang 2011).

Just as health conditions at any time improve with income level, so too, might adverse income shocks have detrimental effects on health. Economic downturns have been linked to increased morbidity and mortality, and to poor nutrition and mental health (societies (Merson, Black and Mills 2012; Lang 2011). The recent economic crisis through the increasing socioeconomic disparities and difficulties such as unemployment, extreme poverty, homelessness, stigma, discrimination and social isolation and through the budgetary constraints and poor policies for financing prevention and treatment, have been translated to heightened risk behaviors on the individual level and impaired public health response on the population level (Paraskevis et al. cited in Economou et al.:101). The negative impacts can also be observed at the societal level, as all sensitive social indicators have been distorted. In European countries, the late 2000's economic crisis laid to a consistent tendency of European governments to diminish the spending on healthcare. This have led to considerable decrease in the number of people accessing healthcare as in countries with weak health insurance policy people had to use money from their pocket (Palascaa and Jabab 2015).

The economic crisis provokes certainly the need for multifactorial adjustments at all health managerial levels. To powerfully address this issue health managers should have clear understanding of the impacts of economic crisis on their ability to maintain and promote an adequate healthcare provision. The present paper will discuss indeed, the main challenges that a health services manager can face regarding the impact of an economic crisis to a local society.

CHAP. 1 : IMPACTS OF AN ECONOMIC CRISIS TO A LOCAL SOCIETY

Given the need for our current society to provide high-quality health care with as wider as possible access, the tight and bidirectional relationship between health status and national income and development has never been too obvious than ever. The health affects income through its direct impact on labor productivity, the extent to which people save their wealth for the future, and age structure. Higher income in turn improves health by increasing the capacity to produce food and have adequate housing and education, and through incentives for planning births (Merson, Black and Mills 2012). So "there is hardly any limit to the ways that economic crisis might affect the health of the population; almost nothing in a modern economy is immune from the effects of economic contraction" (Musgrove 2004:402).

Although the true extent of the health effects of the recent economic crisis is largely unknown, and the lack of systematized studies to clearly monitor the situation (Merson, Black and Mills 2012), there are myriad channels through which an economic crisis may affect human health. First of all, one should consider the case of decline of remuneration or the loss of employment. In 2010, the Greek economy experienced a deep, structural and multi-faceted crisis that spread across all sectors of activity with negative impacts on employment causing an increase in the rate of unemployment which climbed to 27.5% in 2013 (Economou et al.:100). The loss of employment and lower salaries can increase stress and lead to physical and mental health problems including substance abuse, depression, and anxiety. In developing countries with prior poverty background, cases of malnutrition, waterborne diseases and other endemic infectious diseases have just their rates heightened. The subsequent increased health demand in the context of a health system already in financial scarcity create a continuous circuit of chaos (Merson, Black and Mills 2012; Musgrove 2004).

In case of less real income, individuals and households tend to decrease expenditure on essential needs such as the promotion and preservation of health with inadequate adherence to medication regimens, and compromised access to high-quality food or adequate quantities of food which in turn can have immediate and long-term damaging effects particularly on the growth of young children. The Food and Agriculture Organization of the United Nations (FAO) asserts that when a household struggles to cope with economic crises they indirectly put, in one way or another, nutrition and health status of the family at risk (FAO 2009 cited in Merson, Black and Mills 2012). This has been observed at continental level by the famous "austerity measures" set by most European countries in response to the late 2000's economic crisis. The closing down of hospitals and other similar facilities and the lay-offs of medical and supporting personnel or pay cuts had disastrous effects, leading to diminished control over infectious diseases and a lower standard of the services provided (Palascaa and Jabab 2015).

Moreover, fewer financial resources –as consequence of economic crisis- may be available for public health programs during and after times of economic crisis. In Congo (D.R) alike many other developing countries where direct financial supports from the community constitute the most important way sanitary structures are funded (Public Health Ministry 2010), the economic crisis has a special connotation. The heightening of poverty renders the local health system almost inexistent. During the recent economic crisis, high-income countries spent large sums of public money on "bailout" initiatives to the detriment of health and social security. Doing so, the population health becomes more and more vulnerable as public health programs remain unfunded. (Merson, Black and Mills 2012)

CHAP. 2: MAIN MANAGERIAL CHALLENGES IN TIMES OF ECONOMIC CRISIS

As discussed before, the economic crisis has multi-faced consequences since all economic and social sectors are concerned. As a process, Management consists of achieving organizational goals through planning, organizing, directing, and controlling human and physical resources (Swanwick and Mc Kimm 2011, Mokhlis 2011). In time of crisis, carrying out these managerial functions becomes a serious challenge. Successful health care organizations are those that have leaders who understand the nature and implications of external change, and have the ability to set adaptive measures through the development of effective strategies (Ginter, Duncan and Swayne 2013). To efficiently hold the health system through such a difficult period, the manager must call upon his experience to find out all the possible channels by which an economic crisis may affect health and by the way address each of them as separate entity.

To address an economic meltdown some governments tend to diminish the spending on healthcare leading to fewer financial resources available for public health programs during and after times of economic crisis, increased out of pocket payments in some countries, which do not have a robust health insurance policy and a decrease in the number of people accessing healthcare services in the other countries (Palascaa and Jabab 2015, Merson, Black and Mills 2012). In a sensitive sector such as health, the lack of adequate funding and the subsequent reduction of personnel earnings create frustrations that simply melt the devotion of the staff to the vision of the health organization. This leads to failure of the managerial aims as management is the process of getting work done through others (Cummings and Worley 2014:447). Organizing adequate health care provision becomes challenging since lower motivation has negative consequences on the health system performance and renders the managerial processes difficult (Hossein and Vicheth 2011).

To maintain the health sector functioning, the local manager need support both from the public health authorities and the community. Unemployment and lower wages reduce considerably the participation of the society to their own health. This come to say that in economic crises, local managers have to deal with a vulnerable community unable to ensure or pay for their heath; this without sufficient funding from the national level. The resulting financial instability makes the implementation of adaptive measures a tough job. As poverty takes place, cases of malnutrition, waterborne diseases, HIV/AIDS and other endemic infectious diseases have their rates heightened. With the consequent increasing demand for health care, the prior under financed health system can be easily overwhelmed and enter into a total chaos. No manager can be successful with demotivated human resources in a context under financial scarcity.

CONCLUSION

The economic crisis has multi-faced consequences since all economic and social sectors are concerned. This piece of work has discussed the main challenges that a health services manager can face regarding the impact of an economic crisis to a local society. There is tight and bidirectional relationship between health status and national income and development. Just as health conditions improve with income level, so, too, might adverse income meltdown negatively affects health. An economic crisis may affect health through myriads of channels. It increases socioeconomic disparities between people and nations, gives place to diverse social impairments such as unemployment, extreme poverty, homelessness, stigma, discrimination and social isolation. The budgetary constraints and poor policies for financing prevention and treatment have been turned to heightened risk behaviors on the individual level and impaired public health response on the population level. People are constantly exposed to physical and mental health problems including substance abuse, depression, cases of malnutrition, waterborne diseases and other endemic infectious diseases linked to poverty. This come to say that in economic crises, local managers have to deal with a vulnerable community unable to ensure or pay for their heath; this without sufficient funding from the national level. This context of funding scarcity makes the implementation of adaptive measures a tough job. In a sensitive sector such as health, the lack of adequate funding and the subsequent reduction of personnel earnings create frustrations that simply melt the devotion of the staff to the vision ding to the failure of the managerial aims.

No manager can be successful with demotivated human resources in a context under financial scarcity and poverty. So, to efficiently hold the health system through such a difficult period, the manager must call upon his experience to find out all the possible channels by which an economic crisis may affect health and by the way address each of them as separate entity.

BIBLIOGRAPHY

1. Cummings, T. G. Worley, C.G. (2013). *Organization Development and Change.* 10th ed. Mexico, Cengage Learning.
2. Economou, C. Kaitelidou, D. Katsikas, D. et al. "Impacts of the economic crisis on access to healthcare services in Greece with a focus on the vulnerable groups of the population". In *Social Cohesion and Development* 2014 9 (2), 99-115.
3. FAO (Food and Agriculture Organization of the United Nations) (2009). *The state of Food Insecurity in the World: Economic Crises - Impacts and Lessons Learned.* 'Cited in' Merson, M. H., Black, E. R., and Mills, A. J. (2012). *Global Health: Diseases, Programs; Systems and Policies.* 3d ed. London, Jones & Bartlett Learning, LLC.
4. Ginter P. M., Duncan J., Swayne E.L. (2013). *The Strategic Management of Health Care Organizations.* 7th ed. England, John Wiley & sons Ltd.
5. Hossein J. and Vicheth, S. (2011). *Improving Health Sector Performance: Institutions, Motivations and incentive.* Singapore, Institute of Southeast Asian Studies.
6. Lang, R. (2011) "Future challenges to the provision of health care in the 21st century". In: ULC (ed.) *'Consortium of institute of higher education and rehabilitation in Europe Annual conference.* Held 13-15 April 2011, Lisbon: 1-32. Available from ‹ https://www.ucl.ac.uk/lcccr/downloads/presentations/R_LANG_COHEHRE_LISBON_PRESENTATION.pdf›
7. Merson, M. H., Black, E. R., and Mills, A. J. (2012). *Global Health: Diseases, Programs, Systems and Policies.* 3d ed. London, Jones & Bartlett Learning, LLC.
8. Ministry of Public Health (Congo D.R). (2010). *National sanitary plan of development 2011-2015.* Available from ‹http://www.nationalplanningcycles.org/sites/default/files/country_docs/pnds_2011-2015.pdf.› [26-11- 2016].

9. Mokhlis, A. (2011). *Principles of Health Management.* [Online] available from https://me dicalphys.files.wordpress.com/2011/03/lecture-1.ppt [12-9-2016].

10. Musgrove, P. (2004). "Health Economics in Development". In *Human Development Network: Health, Nutrition; and Population Series.* Volume 434. Washington D.C.

11. Palascaa, S. and Jabab, E. (2015) 'Economic crisis' repercussions on European healthcare systems' In *Procedia Economics and Finance* 23 (1) 525 – 533.

12. Paraskevis D, et al., (2013), "Economic recession and emergence of an HIV-1 outbreak among drug injectors in Athens Metropolitan Area: A longitudinal study", *PLoS ONE* 8(11). Cited in Economou, C. Kaitelidou, D. Katsikas, D. et al. "Impacts of the economic crisis on access to healthcare services in Greece with a focus on the vulnerable groups of the population". In Social Cohesion and Development 2014 9 (2), 99-115.

13. Swanwick, T., Mc Kimm, J. (2011). *ABC of clinical Leadership.* Oxford, Wiley-Blackwell.

YOUR KNOWLEDGE HAS VALUE

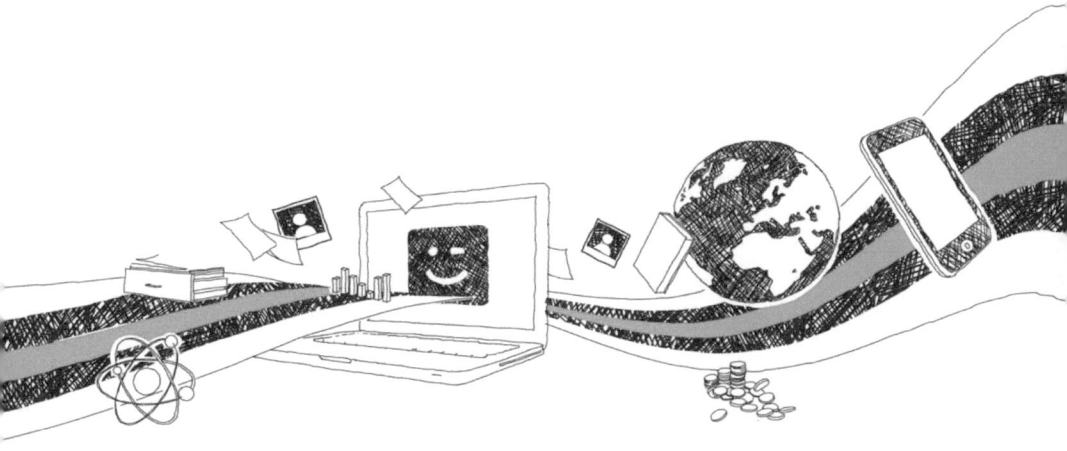

- We will publish your bachelor's and master's thesis, essays and papers

- Your own eBook and book - sold worldwide in all relevant shops

- Earn money with each sale

Upload your text at www.GRIN.com and publish for free